EXERCISING BETWEEN THE SHEETS

A Positive Program for Particular People

By
Don Senecal
With illustrations by Molly Whitney

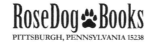

RoseDog🐾Books
PITTSBURGH, PENNSYLVANIA 15238

RoseDog Books
585 Alpha Drive
Suite 103
Pittsburgh, PA 15238
Visit our website at www.rosedogbookstore.com

ISBN: 978-1-4809-7517-0
eISBN: 978-1-4809-7540-8

TABLE OF CONTENTS

ACKNOWLEGEMENTS

I would like to recognize the contributions of Mr. David Zimmerman, professional trainer and student of Pilate, T'ai Chi, and other physical disciplines. David attended Michigan State University studying Exercise Science and Physical Education. His assistance in defining techniques, exercises and the concepts presented here is greatly appreciated. I would also like to thank Ms. Molly Whitney for her splendid illustrations. Keeping it simple and effective. Lastly, I owe my dear wife, Corky a huge thank you for her patience and support during the years of putting this material together. Thanks, Honey!

THE PURPOSE OF THIS BOOK

Now that you have finished giggling about the title of this little book, understand that the intention was to draw your attention and that the book is truly about exercising in bed. Not that sex isn't considered a great form of exercising. Emulating the positions of the Kama Sutra, I understand, is a true physical challenge requiring flexibility and endurance, both wonderful and satisfying elements of a healthy life.

However, what this book will reveal is a wonderful, relaxing and safe way to exercise when the individual's circumstances deny or restrict "normal" avenues of exercising. An alternative to what is generally considered "EXERCISE".

Remember this: Exercise Works. There is no alternative. There is no "quick fix". Exercise, regularly applied and maintained with commitment can result in amazing personal improvements for anyone. The secret is to be honest with yourself and to stay dedicated to yourself and what you want to achieve.

As with any book encouraging physical activity, you should always consult your doctor to determine if this program is suitable for your particular situation.

WHO CAN BENEFIT FROM THIS BOOK?

Here's a hypothetical situation: Suppose there is a person who is considered a "senior citizen", is overweight, has circulatory problems, cannot balance well and has a limited income. This person would not seem to have a very bright future in regards to improving their mobility, flexibility, losing some weight and feeling better. The exercises in this book can help that person significantly improve his or her body strength, coordination, circulation and overall wellness. These personal improvements can take place simply by doing the exercises listed here and slowly increasing the repetitions over an extended period of time.

Be honest. You didn't get to where you are physically over night, did you? Then how could you reasonably expect to lose 30 or 40 pounds and be able to leap tall buildings in just one or two days?

"Exercising Between the Sheets" is considered a reasonable and humane alternative form of exercise and activity that may lead to an improved life style and personal image. Since not all of us can afford or are personally inclined to expose ourselves publicly in more traditional venues of exercise, this book is designed to provide not only a safe and secure place to exercise, but also a variety of exercises that nearly anyone who is alive and breathing can perform. So, who…..?

People who are overweight or may not be able to do deep knee bends, jumping jacks, jogging, power walking or other highly physical exercises:

Of course being overweight is a universal issue. Of course those of us who are overweight know we should do things to look and feel better. Of course all we need is a little "Will Power" and the "Right Program."

If you agree with these statements, you know that it is very easy to say them and very hard to make them a reality. Having a weight challenge is extremely personal. **There is no program or video or book that can make you lose weight unless and until you decide that you need to act. Lastly and always, you are the one who will win the ultimate benefits:**

Maybe you've heard that the TEA Party is an acronym for Taxed Enough Already! I propose that overweight folks consider forming an organization of their own. We could call it the FEA Party (Fat Enough Already!). If being fat were the only criteria, according to recent polls, this new party would have enough members to influence a great deal of what goes on in the world today. Don't think you are alone being fat. People from Friar Tuck to Katherine the Great; from President Taft to Winston Churchill represent only a few famous folks who have faced the challenge of being overweight.

People with physical limitations such as balance issues or may have difficulty getting up and down from the floor.

Not all of us have been blessed with the grace of a gazelle. We stumble, fall or get dizzy from time to time. These situations may be the result of many different conditions, but if you experience them, you know how frustrating and dangerous they can be.

People who have physical challenges such as stability due to disease or accidents or chronic conditions such as Auto-immune issues, Arthritis, Diabetes, etc.:

Something as elementary as an inner-ear infection can effect you regardless of age. Perhaps a car accident or a slip in a bathtub has brought on a situation where your personal stability is in question.

Arthritis, for example, is one of the more prevalent conditions many people must deal with these days. Because the joints suffer from loss of cartilage, they eventually become more difficult to move. Exercise is not impossible, but must be done in a moderate and slowly developing plan to help increase mobility and to strengthen joints. In circumstances like this, it would be wise **(after consulting with your doctor)** to experiment until you find one or two movements that are easiest for you to accomplish without pain. Starting out simply and gradually building as your strength gains is the more reasonable approach. Stretching exercises are a great place to begin because they are low-impact and easily adjusted to your particular needs.

People who may have amputations or partial paralysis:

No matter the cause of paralysis or loss of limbs, movement is a highly recommended process for improving a person's well-being.

People who are self-conscious and do not wish to go to a gym or classes or who just HATE clingy, form-snugging costumes made of material that was never designed to share with the public what you consider extremely private!

How many times have you said to yourself, or heard someone else say, "If I could get in a little better shape first, I wouldn't mind going to a gym". Don't think you are alone in thinking this. Millions of people share your self-consciousness and your reluctance to jump into a revealing body suit or that old pair of sweats to stroll into the local Physical Nirvana Club. Another thing that intimidates many people is the fear of the equipment itself. The staff shows you and demonstrates how easy it is to set speeds on a Treadmill or Stair Stepper, etc. and then you are left alone while they are helping some one else across the building.

People challenged by space itself (or the lack of it) with little or no room for exercise equipment or other paraphernalia:

Many of us live in small apartments next to or above other tenants who do not necessarily appreciate jumping jacks or skipping ropes or mechanical noises. I lived in a downstairs apartment in Los Angeles several years ago. The fellow who lived upstairs exercised with weights. That is, he did until one evening when he dropped one of them and the light over my kitchen table exploded. He never truly "dropped in" on me, but the possibility hung over my head like a black cloud for several months - a very heavy black cloud. Think about the possibilities available to you for exercise in an apartment or small house. Not much. So, you have to be creative and you have to try to be respectful of others living around you as well.

People who have tried "programs" before:

Of course, there's always the "Watch My Beautiful Behind" exercise videos, tapes, programs, etc. If you can afford these things that are sold by the carload to become dust catchers and find them helpful, good for you. Some of us certainly find it difficult to keep up with a lot of media "specialists" who keep urging us to "one more rep"! A lot of these people seem just a little too "perfect" to relate to. In "Between The Sheets" the only person you have to worry about impressing is yourself.

A lot of times, the program accompanies a piece of equipment that may look like a space alien and is "designed to give you the abs you've always dreamed for"! If you've tried them and they work, congratulations. Return this book and get your money back. If you have tried these devices and they are now clothes hangers or yard sale items, let's work out something better.

People who cannot afford expensive programs, personal trainers, physical therapists, coaches, exercise equipment or membership fees to clubs or gyms:

Losing weight and gaining physical fitness can be an expensive issue. Not all of us can afford it. If you add the costs of transportation, "uniforms", dietary supplements, membership dues and fees, etc. – you begin to see why the exercise and weight loss industry makes billions of dollars every year.

People who deal with stress as part of their daily lives:

Regardless of your politics, or your religious beliefs, or your financial condition, or your relational status, today's world continually dumps tons of stress on each and every one of us. We seem to live in an equal-opportunity stress society where we all share collective concerns and personal and professional challenge's as well.

"Between the Sheets" contains specific exercises and routines that will help you relax and cope with the life stresses we encounter on a regular basis.

YOUR EXERCISE PLATFORM

"YOUR BED IS YOUR FRIEND"

What happens in the privacy of your bedroom is your business. It only becomes someone else's business if you choose to make it so.

By utilizing this one piece of furniture in your home that receives the most attention and use, you will be able to attain a level of flexibility and toning that you have not enjoyed for a very long time; a feeling of wellness that may have been denied you simply because you did not have the space or resources or self-motivation.

Your bed is probably the most expensive and well-built piece of furniture you have in your home. It is solid. It is comfortable. It is private. Why shouldn't you be able to use it as you see fit? Why can't you use it to your advantage beyond having it provide a place to rest or read or whatever else you do in there???

Why the bed? Let's be logical. When you're lying down, the stress on your internal organs and your body joints is almost as freeing as being suspended in water. Water exercises for people with certain physical limitations are an excellent way to improve your stamina, muscle strength and flexibility. However, not all of us have access to such an environment. The privacy of your bedroom can be your sanctuary AND your gym.

Not knowing what kind of bed you personally own, all that can be suggested is that it should be firm enough to support you when you exercise. If the mattress is so soft that you sink into it and your spine is distorted, you might try to put a sheet of plywood under it for added support. This book was not written to encourage you to purchase a new mattress, although, if you need one we can't think of a better reason at this time.

Here is a little universal truth…..**doing extremely strenuous exercises is not the only (or even the best in many cases) way to improve your physical condition. The secret of improvement is…moderate exercise on a consistent basis coupled with movement.** By simply moving, your body is forced to react to the needs of your muscles, joints and organs. A person who is inflicted with palsy, a condition where the nerves are constantly stimulated and cause contractions of muscles and muscle groups, is rarely overweight. That is because the body is in constant or nearly constant motion.

Using motion through repetitions, you can achieve improvements. And you can easily do that while laying in bed without worrying if someone notices your larger than life figure or being concerned about falling and breaking a hip.

LETS TALK BENEFITS

Begin a "Benefits List" for yourself. Write them down and look at that list regularly. For the list, consider some of the things you will be able to do better when you exercise on a regular basis. It might be something as mundane as tying your shoes without hearing your ears ring. It might be something as significant as being able to travel across the country to see your family. Sometimes new reasons you haven't considered will show up along the way as you progress. Use some of the following to give you a start. And keep moving!

A basic list of benefits could include:

1. Improved self-confidence.
2. Reduced stress.
3. Improved breathing.
4. More flexibility
5. An improved sense of well-being.
6. Better blood circulation. Improved blood pressure.
7. Better digestion: Lower cholesterol, reduced acid reflux, etc.
8. Better balance.
9. Improved endurance.
10. Improved resistance to colds and infections.
11. Improved functional strength and endurance. "Now I can get

up and down from the floor to play with the grand kids, my pets or spouse"! Now I can carry the groceries from the car to the kitchen!

12. A feeling of accomplishment and personal pride.
13. Feeling well enough to confidently do things like travel, spend time with loved ones (especially any energetic kids you might have in your life), get out without feeling like every trip to the store or park needs to be an ordeal.
14. Have the energy to continue or return to doing things you love like hobbies, sports and more physical pleasures.

Any time you feel yourself falling into a "slump" review these reasons and keep adding more as they occur to you.

TIME FOR AN INSPIRING STORY:

Natalie, when she was in her fifties, woke up one day to "suddenly" find she was overweight, not strong enough to complete many of her former daily activities and had been diagnosed with a host of health issues including orthopedic problems and fibromyalgia – a chronic condition that manifests itself in aching muscles and extremely low energy levels. One of the tricky things about dealing with fibromyalgia, Natalie found, was that if she did too little activity, she was very tired and sore and if she did too much, she was also tired and sore. Through careful experimentation, Natalie found the right formula and keeps making adjustments as her physical condition improves. The "Moral" of the story? Keep trying; make adjustments; keep up the good effort.

NUMBER ONE EXERCISE: BREATHING

Try this: Lie on your back in a comfortable position and EXHALE as far as possible, then relax. See? Your body automatically breathes in when it needs air. It's how nature fills a void.

Breathing is the essential exercise. The average person uses about 50% capacity of their lungs. Since oxygen is the basic "fuel" of life it needs to be replenished and cleansed regularly. The more you exert yourself, the more oxygen your body requires to work efficiently. Before and during your exercises, be sure to take time to breath deeply.

How we breathe has a major effect on our exercise and our health. In fact, in the Chinese practice of Tai Chi, we are considered to get our energy in only two ways: eating food and breathing.

Ultimately, we want the body to breathe naturally, but sometimes years of bad habits, stress, poor posture, physical challenges, etc. get in the way. When we're exercising, often the breath will get more rapid and change in its qualities. This is natural, and we don't want to get in the way of that. However, you will find it useful to be aware of the breath at nearly all times during exercises and on the breaks in between. This can be a terrific way to have a good sense of what's going on with your body today, in the present moment.

Next, take in five, slow breaths, taking in as much air as you possibly can and then exhaling as thoroughly as you are able. Repeat this exercise between each exercise group that you complete during your work-out period. Notice that we refer to breathing as an exercise. The lungs need flexibility to adapt to the added demand for oxygen that your movements will create.

As you breathe, place your hand gently on your stomach. You should feel it going up and down. This is breathing properly and it isn't goofy. It is called Diaphragmatic Breathing or Belly Breathing. Watch any baby sleeping on its back and you will see that natural breathing is belly breathing.

Done regularly as an exercise, you can actually expand the capacity and flexibility of your lungs.

NUMBER TWO EXERCISE: CONTRACTION AND RELAXATION

In the Wizard of Oz[1], there's a scene where Dorothy and the Straw Man come upon the Tin Woodsman who happens to be rusted into a frozen position. While trying to help, they hear the Tin Man murmur, "Oil can! Oil can!" The Straw Man says, "Oil can what?" (Which is a pretty funny line!). Dorothy realizes that what is needed is the oil from the can to lubricate the Tin Mans' joints and the show goes on from there.

One of the traditional signs the medical community associates with aging is a reduction in the elasticity of the bodies various tissues. That is to say our tissue's natural ability to expand and contract is lessened. Muscles can become tight and cause stress on the joints. Blood vessels harden and provide less effective circulation. Soft tissue in the joint "dries out" and becomes compressed. Please don't think that WD-40 is in order here!

An advantage of exercising in the way presented here is that you can emphasize not just contraction, but relaxation as well. Just like breathing in needs breathing out, a healthy body requires the ability to both contract and expand. These are both skills that we can learn and improve.

---

[1] 1939 Film produced by MGM

RESULTS AND EXPECTATIONS – TAKING CHARGE OF YOUR OWN BODY AND YOUR OWN CHALLENGES.

Let's face it. Not everyone has access to a local gym or swimming pool or personal trainer or exercise equipment. Not everyone can afford the time or money to regularly attend classes at the local recreation facility or commercial gym in order to keep in shape. And certainly, a lot of us have "expanded" beyond the Spandex generation! Many of us have restrictions in our funds, our time and our ability to be mobile.

Being self-conscious about how we look or feel matters first and foremost to ourselves alone. No one except you can do what needs to be done, so please:

1. Be kind to yourself. If you pause once in a while for a day or so, don't think of yourself as a failure. It's just a break in the activity and you will get back to it with an added energy and determination.
2. Practice tough love on yourself. Stress not thinking of yourself as a loser. Talk openly with yourself about what you need to do to accomplish significant and noticeable improvements.

Swearing is ok if you're used to it. If not, no need to start.

3. Encourage yourself. Remember the benefits we listed earlier and review them constantly. Good things are what you want to focus on.

4. Give yourself credit for every step along the way. When you lose some weight, be happy. When you can open a jar that you were unable to handle before, be proud of your progress. Don't be afraid to pat yourself on the back.

NO ONE IS EVEN GOING TO PRETEND THIS IS EASY. But no one else is better situated to help you succeed. Talking to and encouraging yourself is perfectly permissible. I talk to myself all the time and my wife has only questioned it once or twice, honest!

Another point to be emphasized is: **Don't think you won't try to rationalize yourself out of doing this stuff.** It's so easy to say, "I'm feeling tired today, I deserve a break". But what is it you are really saying to yourself? Are you saying you deserve not to do the work or that you deserve to never have the benefits? When you start to do that, try to remember –if you don't put in the work, you can't enjoy the rewards.

GOOD TO KNOW

Instant gratification expectations do not work! Just like, "Lord, grant me patience (and I want it RIGHT NOW!)". Twenty years of experience tells me that those who work and realize short-term results do not maintain them. Lose 20 pounds in a month and odds are in two months you will have them back plus a couple for "bad measure". Take your time – don't think that by doing 20 reps in 10 seconds constitutes exercising. What is suggested here is that you have a chance to commit to realistic, gradual and permanent change. **Give yourself some time**.

Another inspirational story: A person we know had smoked all their lives and was struggling with quitting. They realized what was at stake, but couldn't make much progress. It seems that after a week or so, they'd go back to smoking and when they did, friends and family would criticize and generally make life hell. They felt like the world's biggest loser because they lacked the will power to quit. Then this person happened to move to Italy for about a year because of work. In Italy people didn't judge or condemn, they actually offered this person cigarettes! All of a sudden, this person didn't feel like a failure or a loser because they didn't feel they were being judged or criticized by others. A "no thank you" to offers for cigarettes became natural and quitting became a much easier thing to accomplish.

PREPARATION

PLAN YOUR ROUTINE

Being consistent with any kind of exercise is a good thing. It helps to plan your day and to anticipate what can become part of your daily routine. It also helps you mentally prepare yourself as well as being part of a modest discipline in your life. I would suggest the following:

Consider what time of day you feel most comfortable doing your exercises. If you are a morning person, then the stretches and flexes will help you loosen up and energize you for the day ahead. If you prefer later in the day, that's fine too only try not to do your routines just before trying to sleep. Give yourself a little time to wind down and relax. Do you want to work with the lights on or off, the windows open or closed, etc.? Remember, you need to feel comfortable and secure before you begin and during the exercise time. Try to plan your exercises when there will be no interruptions or distractions.

Block out a period of time. Be realistic. The goal is 20 to 30 minutes (at a minimum) each day to do your exercises. However, if 10 to 15 or even 5 to 10 minutes is a comfortable starting period for you, then that's where you start. This time could be early or late in the day, but you should do it consistently. Stay with your program!

Turn off the phone, computer, television, radio, cell phone and any other electronic or mechanical devices that may distract. If you find that music helps, then by all means pick out something that will support your activity and go for it!

Suggestion: Get yourself an inexpensive egg-timer. One of my biggest frustrations when exercising is to set a goal of twenty minutes and then constantly looking at the clock like "Are We There Yet?" A timer is something you don't have to think about and it will let you know when you're "there"!

Take a moment to set your expectations for your exercises on any given day. This can be helped by using an exercise log. A sample of one is included in this book.

Begin by lying on your back with your body in a spread-eagle position. This is the primary position from which most of these exercises begin.

Be sure you have freedom of movement and have removed any obstructions such as binding clothes or heavy blankets, etc.

Now that you have made your plans, remember, that as your own personal trainer, you have the prerogative of changing the rules! Whatever happens, you must promise yourself to make an honest effort.

We're sure you're just itching to begin with the hard-core stuff. The only problem is that there isn't any! What we're asking you to do is to start out slowly with a great deal of patience. Don't force your body to do anything it's not ready to do. TAKE YOUR TIME! Understand how long it may have taken to get where you are physically and that to reverse and improve will also take time plus effort. In an age where instant gratification is the mantra of society, it may be frustrating for a while, but every time you purposely move a finger, flex a muscle, bend a joint or take a deep breath, you are making progress.

EXERCISES

FIRST SERIES:
STRETCHING AND BUILDING MOVES

Stretching is essential for keeping the muscles loose and free-flowing. It allows the blood to circulate more readily and it can be a relaxing as well as invigorating way to exercise. Think of the family cat or dog when they first get wake up and do those really loooong stretches.

1. Frog stroke: Beginning with the feet and legs together and straight, pull the heels of your feet towards your behind while keeping your legs on the bed. Imagine how a frogs legs look when they swim. As you start to pull your knees apart, your feet bottoms should come together. Straighten your legs. Relax and repeat.

2. Lying with your legs together, pull the left knee towards your left side (waist) without raising your leg from the bed (just like the frog-leg thing in number 1) while bringing your heel towards your behind. Straighten the left leg and then pull the right knee towards your right side while keeping your leg on the bed. Straighten the right leg. Repeat, alternating left and right legs. **NOTE:** This is just like #1 except with one leg at a time.

3. Special "Guns": (Note: this exercise requires one or two cans of soup [unopened is preferred!]). Holding a can of soup in each hand and having your arms lying on the bed, palms up next to your body, lift one arm, bending at the elbow towards your shoulder. Alternate each arm "curl".

4. The Great Arm Lift: Extend both arms straight out from the shoulders and keep them on the bed and spread your legs to about shoulder width for a "Spread-Eagle" look. Now, with or without soup cans in your hands (we suggest starting out without them), bring your arms up to bring the palms together above your face trying to touch the ceiling.

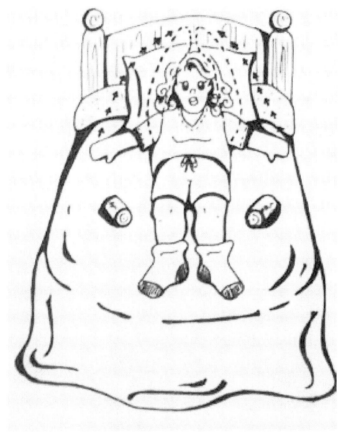

#4 The Great Arm Lift

5. Arm Reaching: Laying your hands with the palms flat on the bed, raise the left arm all the way to over your head so that it is lying on the bed (you may have to move toward the foot of the bed to accommodate this move). Bring the left arm back down to your side. Do the same movement with your right arm. Repeat, alternating left and right. Note: You can do this exercise with soup cans too.

6. Leg Slides: Keeping your legs together and stretched straight, pull one foot back towards your buttocks, keeping your foot flat on the bed as it slides. Straighten the leg and repeat with the other leg.

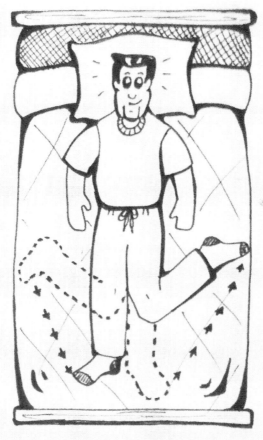

#6 Leg Slides

7. Head Twist: While pointing your chin at the ceiling, slowly turn your head to the left and point your chin at your left shoulder. Bring your head back to center, then turn to the right and point your chin at your right shoulder. Try to get your ear flat to the bed. Repeat.

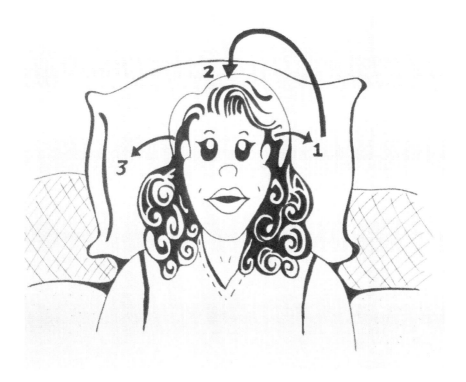

#7 Head Twist

8. Rolling Legs: While spreading your arms straight out from your sides and keeping your legs straight, roll slightly to your left and drag your right leg over your left leg to where your right leg is nearly at 90 degrees to your hips. Bring the right leg back to straight and roll to the right while doing the same movement with the left leg. Repeat.

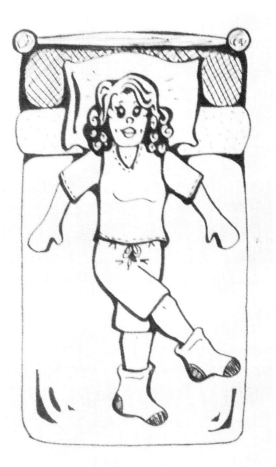

#8 Rolling Legs

9. Rolling Arms: While spreading your arms straight out from your sides and keeping your legs straight, bring your right arm up and over your body while rolling to your left. Try to touch the fingers of both hands. Bring you right arm back to the original position and then bring the left arm up and over while rolling to your right. Try to touch the fingers of both hands. Bring the left arm back to the original position. Repeat.

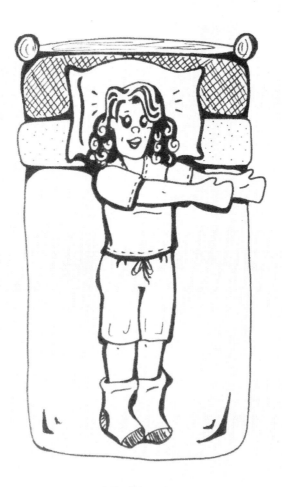

#9 Rolling Arms

10. Wrist Bending: With your fingers together and pointed at the ceiling at arms length, bend your wrist down and back. Do this back and forth slowly like waving with both hands together. Repeat.

11. Leg Spreads. With knees straight and toes pointed at the ceiling, spread your legs as far apart as possible. Hold for a slow count to 5, relax. Repeat.

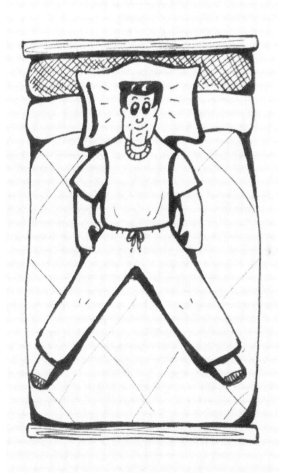

#11 Leg Spreads

12. Leg Dangles: Move down the bed until your legs are dangling over the edge of the mattress at the knees. Beginning with the left leg, straighten the leg at the knee until it is level with your thigh and body. Lower the leg and do the same movement with the right leg. Alternate.

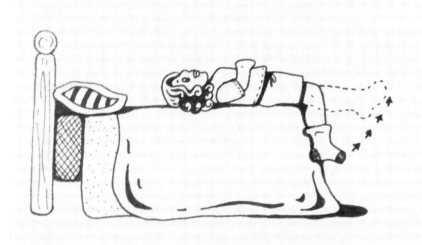

#12 Leg Dangles

13. Lay on the left side with your head resting on your left palm. Place your right palm flat on the mattress in front of your chest. Lift your right leg as high as possible for a count of 5 and then lower the leg. Repeat for 10 to 20 reps. Turn over onto your right side, with the alternate hands in the same position and lift the left leg for a count of 5. Repeat for 10 to 20 reps.

14. While lying on your left side as in exercise number 13, extend your right arm straight in front of you. Spread the fingers of your right hand as wide as possible and swing you arm backwards as far as possible and hold for a count of 5. Bring the arm back to the front position and repeat the back and forth motion for 10 to 20 reps. Turn onto your right side and repeat the same movements with the left arm.

15. While in the beginning position for exercise 13, with your right arm extended straight in front of you, swing your arm from front to back. Turn onto your right side and repeat the same movements with the left arm.

16. While in the beginning position for exercise 13, extend your right arm down the length of your side. Raise the arm straight up and over your head to touch the headboard or wall. Bring the arm back down to your side. Repeat. Turn onto your right side and repeat the same movements with the left arm.

17. Body stretches. (Watch animals) This exercise is as simple as waking in the morning. Just stretch out your entire body and arch your back a little and enjoy that first stretch of the morning feeling. If you have not done this for some time, we guarantee you will enjoy it!

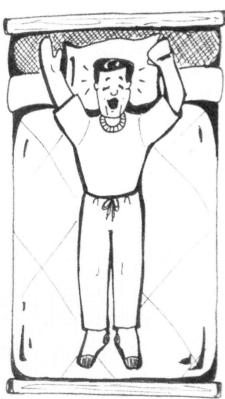

#17 Body Stretches

BREAK TIME

How should it feel when you're working out at an appropriate intensity? A helpful skill that many of us need to learn is how to distinguish the difference between "pain" and "discomfort". This book does not subscribe to the philosophy of "no pain-no gain". Pain is our body's way of telling us something is wrong, and it should be listened to.

Discomfort, unlike pain, can be a way that our body is telling us it's learning or experiencing something new. In order to get stronger, we need to put our bodies into new situations and there may be a level of discomfort that accompanies that. A burning sensation in a muscle; a general feeling of fatigue; a moderate straining, these are all natural, healthy sensations.

Pain may come in the form of feelings like "tearing", "crunching", or sharp sensations at the joint site. These are all sensations you want to give a great amount of respect. If you experience any of these signs: back off, slow down, modify, or stop the exercise altogether.

Let's talk cramps:

Cramps hurt like heck (and sometimes much more!). Everyone gets cramps from time to time. It is part of life's cycle and is to be expected. If you suffer from frequent or severe cramping, talk to your Doctor. Muscle cramps we refer to here are those that might result from exercise.

A cramp is the involuntary contraction of a muscle or set of muscles that result in temporary immobility and pain. The most common example would be the good 'ol (or bad 'ol) Charlie Horse. Why they decided to call it Charlie, I don't have a clue, but when the calf of your leg tightens up and feels like a horse has just bit you, you know exactly what a cramp is and how it feels!

Muscle cramps are usually caused by loss of fluid or over-activity (stressing muscles and muscle groups).

The best way to treat a muscle cramp is to prevent it from happening in the first place. In order to do that, remember two things:

1. Drink plenty of water. 2. Be sure to warm up your muscles gradually and stretch well afterwards. If you DO experience a cramp, there are some things you can do to ease the pain:

1. Try stretching the muscle by flexing or walking around on it a little
2. Rub it vigorously.
3. Apply some warmth to the area with a heating pad or hot water bottle, etc.

Cramps usually last for only a few moments – it only feels like years. If you continue to experience cramps while trying to exercise on a regular basis, stop and consult your doctor.

Another Inspirational Story – Goal Setting – Staying on Track:
Tom, in his 40s, while many folks are just coming into the "top" of their game career-wise, as parents, and having the resources and abilities to participate fully in their favorite activities, Tom went to the hospital with very serious flu-like symptoms. What was happening, Tom found out was that he was having a brain-stem stroke, where the blood and oxygen are cut off from a part of the brain that is responsible for many of our basic, life-sustaining functions. Months later Tom rolled out of the hospital in a wheelchair and went home with his wife and two young children with a determination that reminds one of the Teddy Roosevelt quote: "Do what you can with what you have where you are". A lot of traditional exercise goals weren't of much use to Tom, but at one point his mantra became to accomplish a "first" every day. On a good day, it might be transferring from the bed to the wheelchair with assistance. On a more challenging day, it might be breath meditation that he had never tried before. Tom found a way to commit completely to his own well being while making room for working with and through any stumbling blocks along the way. Today, Tom continues to improve,

living with a condition which many people are never able to leave a facility. Tom works a full-time job, is a fantastic father of two college students, has a rich home life, spends time in the out-of-doors and continues to fill his days with many "firsts".

SECOND SERIES: FLEXES

If you watch body builders on television or see them on the covers of magazines at the grocery store, you know that they "strike poses" and flex to show off their muscles. What they are doing is tightening muscle groups in a planned way to show off their best assets. What you will be doing here is doing what they do…flexing individual muscles or groups of muscles. You don't need to break out the body oil yet. Besides, you might just slide out of bed!

Unless otherwise instructed, all exercises are done while lying on your back in the middle of the bed.

1. Toe curls: Bring back your toes, trying to point them at your knees, then, curling your toes and tensing your calves, point you toes away from your knees as far as possible. Hold for a count of 5 and relax. Repeat.
2. Stomach flexes: Tighten your stomach muscles just as though you were expecting your ugly, obnoxious 8 year old nephew to hit you in the stomach. Hold for a count of 5 and relax. Repeat.
3. Butt crunch: Tighten your buttocks, squeezing the cheeks together. Relax and repeat.
4. Fist-Springs: Lift your arms until you are looking up at the backs of your hands. Now squeeze them tightly into balled fists.

Then pop them open with fingers wide spread (so they look surprised). Repeat.

5. Stomach Crunchies: While flexing your stomach as in exercise two, lift you head off the bed and try to see your toes. Hold for a count of 5 and relax. Repeat.

6. Shoulder Squeeze: While pointing your chin at the ceiling, bring your shoulders up to touch your ears (this may not work, but if your ears are as big as mine, you may have a shot!). Hold for a count of 5 and relax. Repeat.

7. Shoulder Drop: While tucking your chin (make a double chin), pull your shoulder blades down towards your behind. Keep your stomach muscles firm as well. Hold for a count of 5 and relax. Repeat.

8. Elbowing the Bed: With your elbows on the bed and your hands towards the ceiling (90 degrees at elbows), flex your upper back muscles to push your elbows into the bed (try not to raise your shoulders towards your ears). Hold for a count of 5 and relax. Repeat.

9. Picking on the Pecs: While pointing your chin at the ceiling, tighten your chest muscles (imagine you are one of those muscle-bound beach boys striking a pose). Hold for a 5 count and relax. Repeat.

10. The Runaway Calf and Thunder Thighs Flex: Concentrate on the calves and thighs and slowly flex them to a tight bundle. Hold for a count of 5 and relax. Repeat.

12. The "Whole package" flex. While doing the various muscle group flexes, you may have noticed that other groups got involved along the way. When you were tightening up the legs, you felt the stomach needing to join in. Once you have moved through the individual groups, feel free to try to involve as much of the entire body in the muscle tightening; having the whole body go rigid for a few moments and then relaxing.

NOTE: Be sure to go through the entire list before you do the whole body thing because controlling various muscle groups individually is great for the concentration and body control. It also improves balance and stability.

BONUS BUNDLE ONE

Facial Exercises:

In the world of acting and public speaking, there are a number of facial exercises that are encouraged to keep the neck and mouth and tongue muscles flexible and strong. The following exercises are simple, but effective. Try them for a few days and you will actually feel the difference.

1. Chin Thrust. Like an aggressive Drill Sergeant barking orders, shove your lower jaw into a lower teeth-jutting scowl. You Bulldog you. Relax and repeat.

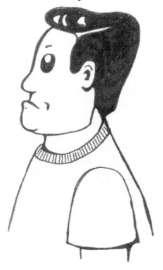

#1 Chin Thrust

2. Cheshire Grin. Make the biggest grin with your lips together possible.

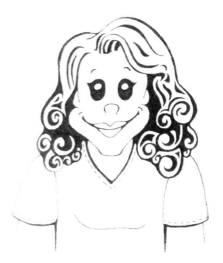

#2 Cheshire Grin

3. Grin and sniff it. While doing the Cheshire grin, wrinkle up your nose.

4. Lion's Roar. Try to touch your chin with your tongue with your mouth as open as possible.

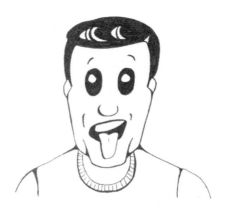

#4 Lion's Roar

5. Kiss Kiss. While laying on your back, try to kiss the ceiling

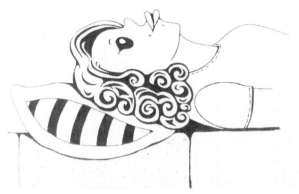

#5 Kiss Kiss

6. The big pout. Try to cover your upper lip with your lower lip. Just like when you were 5 (or yesterday, if it applies).

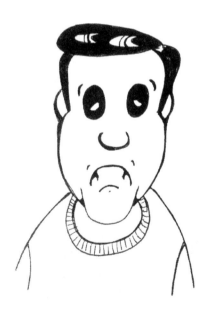

#6 The Big Pout

7.   The Gold Fish. While keeping your lips together, draw in your cheeks.

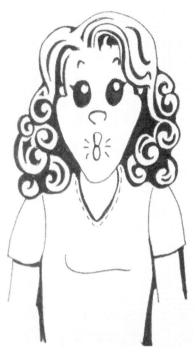

#7 The Gold Fish

8.   Face Scruntch. While pulling down your eyebrows, scruntch up your nose, close your eyes and squint. This is a kind of face you'd make sucking on a lemon.

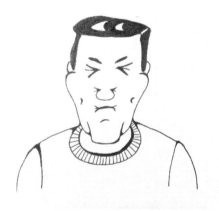

#8 Face Scruntch

9. The Surprise Party. Open your eyes and mouth as wide a possible while raising your eyebrows. Everyone should be yelling, "Surprise!"

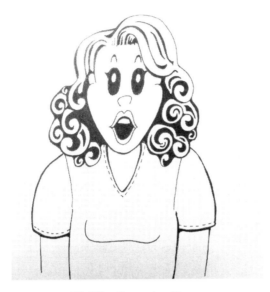

#9 The Surprise Party

One bit of advice about these exercises. Although they are known to be of benefit to the muscles of your face, mouth and neck, do not do them while looking into a mirror or in front of the children. You will laugh and they might cry.

BONUS BUNDLE TWO

EXERCISE YOUR BRAIN:

This might seem like a silly suggestion, but you need to pay attention (because that's a good way to exercise the brain!). Besides which, when was the last time you ever read about somebody pulling a "Brain tendon" or "rupturing their cortex"?

What I'm suggesting here is finding ways to engage your brain ("the little grey cells" as Hercule Poirot[2] would say) in a kind of exercise to stimulate and engage the thought process as well as the more physical muscles of the body. There are many excellent "exercises" to challenge your thought processes. Some of which are pretty common such as working crossword puzzles or Zudoko. Those are in the daily paper and are very good. Beyond that, there are more creative challenges such as video games, reading a good book or hobbies such a putting those little ships in bottles and there are "brain exercises on line as well. Going even further, you could try denying yourself one of your senses for a period of time and forcing your other senses to compensate:

1. Close your eyes while trying to dress yourself.
2. Take a different route to work or the store.
3. Re-arrange the furniture.
4. Use your sense of touch to navigate through your living space.

---

[2] A Detective character of Agatha Christie

By keeping your eyes closed, you are challenging other senses to help you be aware of your surroundings. The placement of objects like chairs and tables and doors to other rooms become a challenge to the sense of touch.

5. Pay attention to the smell of your food or when you are out and about, the odor of flowers or if you are passing a dairy farm. Trust me, your nose will alert you to many interesting things! The sense of smell is said to trigger more memories than all of the others combined.

All of these small things enable your brain to act more creatively and allows you to respond in a much more primitive and basic way to your environment. It also creates new patterns of connections within your brain which stimulates your "mental visual perspective". These are all good things for you and your brain.

RECORD KEEPING

The most important thing about these exercises is - **DO THEM!** If you have limited time and your choice is to document or do, always choose do. Documentation, however, is a wonderful way to chart your progress, assess whether your routine is working well for you, head off possible problems and get an objective measure of things.

The following is a sample exercise log that includes some ways to track your workouts.

Date					
Breathing Exercise					
Contraction/Relaxation Exercise					
Series 1: Flexes					
1. Toe Curls					
2. Stomach Flexes					
3. Butt Crunch					
4. Fisti-Springs					
5. Stomach Crunchies					
6. Shoulder Squeeze					
7. The Shoulder Drop					
8. Elbowing the Bed					
9. Picking on the Pecs					
10. Runaway Calf and Thunder Thighs					
11. The Whole Package					

Series 2: Stretching and Building					
1. Frog Stroke					
2. Frog Stroke 2					
3. Special "Guns"					
4. The Great Arm Lift					
5. Arm Reaching					
6. Leg Slides					
7. Head Twist					
8. Rolling Legs					
9. Rolling Arms					
10. Wrist Bending					
11. Leg Spreads					
12. Leg Dangles					
13. Leg Heft					
14. Arm Stretch					
15. Big Wave					
16. Back Stroke					
17. Body Stretches					

Bonus Bundle 1: Facial Exercises					
1. Chin Thrust					
2. Chesire Grin					
3. Grin and Sniff It					
4. Lion's Roar					
5. Kiss Kiss					
6. The Big Pout					
7. The Gold Fish					
8. Face Scruntch					
9. The Surprise Party					
Bonus Bundle 2: Exercise Your Brain(place a "check" if completed)					
1. Closed Eyes Dressing					
2. Different Route					
3. Re-Arrange					
4. Touch Navigation					

My Energy Level Today (1-10)					
My Workout Felt ___ (1-10)					
My Greatest Success Today					
(place a "#" and record on back)					
Notes: (place an "*" and record on back)					

OTHER GOOD STUFF TO KNOW

How often should I exercise? The recommendation is to set aside time each day, but as you will learn, a lot of these exercises can be done while you are watching TV or taking a bath, etc. The Facial gymnastics in Bonus Bundle One are possible anywhere so if you can sneak in a few extra reps while reading the paper, do it!

What you eat and drink
Any exercise program will be very limited in the results department if you're not addressing things from the nutritional side as well. If you are not an expert on nutrition, we recommend educating yourself on what a healthy diet for you looks like. There are many great books available as well as many qualified dieticians. If you can't afford private service, call your local city or county health department and ask for help. Tapping these resources to learn more will pay for itself over and over in your life.

Eating a sound, healthy diet is the best policy. Fortunately, there are some very simple, general guidelines that you can follow that may help. It's no secret that Americans eat way too much processed food and fast food. These are both practices that can seriously reduce the effect of all the work you're putting in with your exercise program.

In the same way that we suggest that you consult with your doctor before beginning any exercise program, we would also suggest that you consult with a nutritionist or your doctor before dieting.

Here's a list of some helpful principles:

1. Eat lots of fresh vegetables and fruits.
2. Prepare your own food as much as possible.
3. Find out what a proper portion size is for you based on your size and activity level (here's where a nutritionist comes in handy).
4. Eat food from the produce and meat counters, not the places where everything is in boxes (this stuff has "additives" and chemicals that may not be so good for you).
5. Read the labels on packages you do buy. Avoid products that use words like "Hydrogenated, hydrolyzed, corn syrup and high fructose corn syrup".
6. Eat good, quality foods that you enjoy, not foods that are supposed to be "good for you".
7. Eat slowly (this is a big challenge for most of us who always seem to be in a hurry!). Allow yourself time to savor the flavors and breathe between bites. Try not to watch TV or read while eating. Maybe listen to relaxing music instead.
8. Drink 8-10 glasses of water a day. (see the section about water further on in the book).
9. Limit "drinking" your calories, especially in the form of alcohol and sugary drinks.
10. Educate yourself about different types of calories (protein, fat, and carbohydrates)
11. Educate yourself about the difference between "good fats" and "bad fats". Concentrate on eating some of the good ones and limiting the baddies. Do the same with carbohydrates as well.

12. Allow yourself occasional "cheat dates" and enjoy some of your favorite foods that may not be on your "balanced diet" list. Remember, we are in this for the long haul, not the short sprint!

The simplest way we can state nutrition and diet action for you is to **STOP EATING JUNK AND KEEP MOVING!** If you don't know the difference between junk food and good food, ask for help!

DRINKING PLENTY OF WATER – THE WHY AND WHEREFORE

When you exercise, your body does more than just use up water. That is not why you need to drink plenty of it. What happens is that when you exercise, chemical things happen in your muscles, good things like they get little, tiny tears in them and after you stop exercising, it takes a little time for those little tears to heal BUT when they heal, they heal stronger with more muscle tissue than fat. So, why the water? When you exercise and tear your muscles (in a good way) it also releases bad chemicals and those need to be flushed out of your system. That's why you need to drink the water, not because you are thirsty (although you may very well be), but to flush out the bad stuff and to assist in the healing and building of your muscles. How much should you drink? The recommended standard for an adult is between 8 to 12 eight ounce glasses of water each day. Of course, don't get carried away with this. I don't want you wetting the bed and blaming the book!

A FINAL SALUTE

What you have committed to doing as a result of purchasing and reading this book is an admirable thing. You have decided that you want to improve your life and to enjoy living to the best of your ability. I hope that you have enjoyed reading the material and that you also enjoy applying the principles and dynamics of this book to your own life style and that the results prove to be both positive and beneficial. When that happens, you have completely made my day!

SOMETHING ABOUT ME…

Let me tell you a little about myself so you will be filled with awe and wonder at my marvelous backgrounds, education, experience and ability to completely change your lives……or just to know me better!

I was born and raised in Vancouver, Washington. I grew up a country boy but eventually wound up receiving a Master's Degree in Communicative Arts from the University of Portland. For 20 years I worked as a Recreation Professional in Vancouver and Tacoma, Washington. My emphasis has always been on well-being and enjoyment of life. Through coordinating senior citizen classes and activities to art, dance, movement and martial arts classes, every attempt has been to improve the life experience. Being semi-retired, my wife Corky and I now live (with our little dog Zoey), work and play in beautiful Bend, Oregon where golf, hiking, camping and fishing beckon.